LOW CARB CHAFFLE COOKBOOK

Quick And Easy Healthy Recipes For Your Everyday Meals

AMBER WOOLERY

Low Carb Chaffle Cookbook

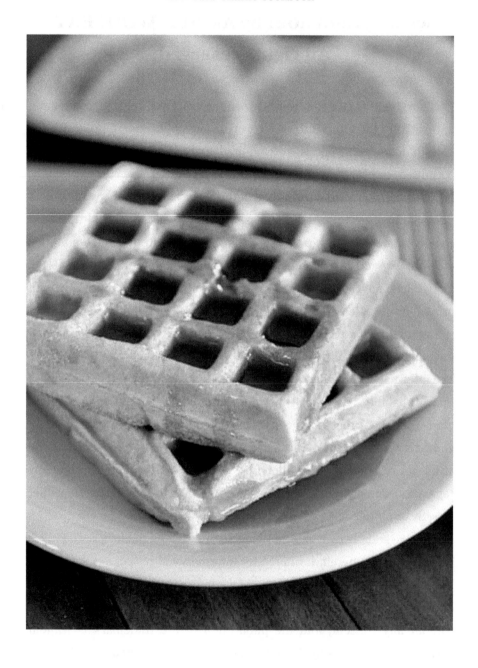

Table of Contents

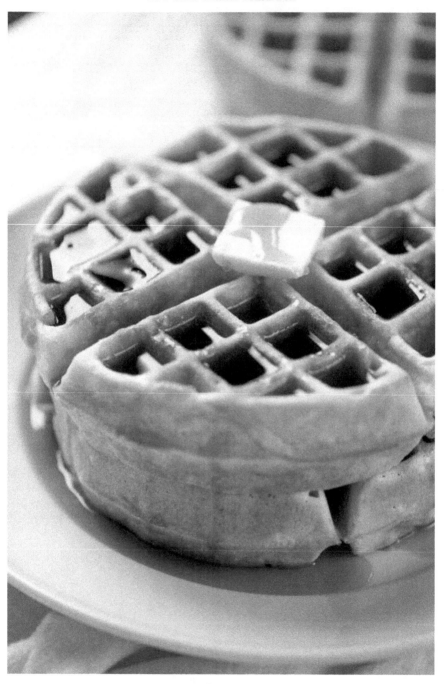

Introduction

If you're on a ketogenic diet or contemplating one, you're aware that certain ingredients are off-limits. This is due to their carbohydrate content. The aim of the diet is to bring your body through ketosis, where it burns fat rather than carbohydrates for energy. The ketosis phase will not begin if you consume too many carbohydrates.

That means eliminating all carbohydrates, beans, and most sugar from your diet and replacing them with fat from foods like eggs, yogurt, cheese, coconut oil, avocados, and other healthy fats.

Since the keto diet has been around for a while, there are several creative people out there creating keto-friendly versions of just about every treat you can think of.

Waffles are delicious. Waffles come in a range of varieties, so it's easy to choose one that you like. Alternatively, you might develop a whole different taste.

Take a traditional waffle, put something extra on top, or tweak the batter slightly, and you've created a new waffle! So, what if you're on a ketogenic diet?

How do you enjoy the waffles now?

The chaffle is the answer!

Chaffles are delicious on their own, with a distinct flavor.

The chaffle is a waffle without the grain because it's one of those sweets. The chaffle will help you fulfill your cravings for comfort foods while on the keto diet, particularly bread.

There are ample types, much like traditional waffles, for everyone to find a liking.

This book aims to immerse the audience in the chaffle-making method. To serve as a resource for anything related to this process. And, ideally, it would succeed. So, switch the page and get rolling! The chaffles are set to be prepared and fed!

CHAPTER 1:

Basics of Keto Diet

A ketogenic diet usually has a 15:4:1 fat, protein, and carbohydrate ratio. When anyone follows the keto diet, they are automatically drawn to more proteins, which is why many people refer to it as a high-protein diet. The Atkins diet is a form of ketogenic eating plan. Counting carbohydrates is essential on the Atkins diet. The conventional ketogenic diet, on the other side, promotes fat intake.

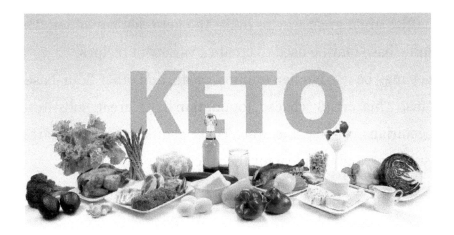

The end aim of a ketogenic diet is to reprogram your body to enter ketosis. If the body doesn't have enough glucose, it does this. The key component in starchy foods and sugars is glucose. When the body breaks down fat, it releases ketones, which are acids. Obese people can feel compelled to consume still more calories. As a result, this lifestyle is ideal for them since it keeps one complete for longer.

You should check the scent of your breath to see if your body is in a ketosis state. Ketones are notorious for giving off a fruity odor that can be found in your air. You must be mindful that you will be reducing your glucose intake. As a result, you can eat nutritious foods to maintain your fitness.

Consuming proteins such as seafood, beef, milk, dairy, poultry, and cheese are examples of these commodities. Ghee, butter, plant-based oils, and other naturally derived fats are all healthy choices.

Chaffles are a great way to make the keto diet smoother. The chaffle base may be used to create a variety of recipes.

They may be used in lieu of buns, pasta, and other flour-based items. This crispy cheese foundation is a great substitute. Vegetarians will like it as well. These chaffles are low in carbs, taste great, and are ideal for the keto diet.

Ketogenic Diet - Health Benefits

The keto diet has many health advantages. It will assist you with being more involved and successfully controlling your blood sugar levels. The aim is to get through ketosis and burn more fat for energy. Let's look at some of the keto diet's nutritional advantages.

Helps in weight loss

As previously said, the keto diet aids weight loss by preventing the body from producing adequate glucose, which causes the body's fat metabolism to begin. Fat is the body's energy storage medium, and its dissolution results in weight loss. Many diets for weight reduction that you might have followed have failed, and you are starving. The keto diet, on the other side, is more apt to help you feel healthy during the day.

Reduces Acne

Acne may be attributed to the body's blood sugar level. When your body is in a ketosis condition, your blood sugar level is relatively poor, which ensures your acne may be regulated, and in certain instances, it can even go away entirely.

Reduce Risk of Cancer

There are several research trials and inquiries into the effects of a ketogenic diet on cancer prevention. Since it is said to induce a high degree of oxidative stress in cancer cells, it is being used instead of chemotherapy. It may also help to control blood glucose levels and may help to prevent diabetes problems that are also associated with cancer.

Improves heart health

If you adopt the keto diet in a safe manner, you have a fair chance of boosting your heart's condition and lowering the risk of heart attacks. This is because eating healthy fats like avocados while using plant-based oils will help you raise HDL cholesterol while lowering LDL cholesterol.

Reduces Seizures

The keto diet's efficacy in preventing epilepsy is the subject of a lot of studies. However, in certain instances, the diet has resulted in a decline or, in some circumstances, a complete cessation of seizures. This therapy is said to be very effective in children, particularly those who suffer from focal seizures.

Increases brain function

When you switch to a keto diet, your brain capacity is said to improve dramatically. It's claimed to have a slew of neural advantages. Any individuals with Parkinson's disease have reported that following a ketogenic diet has improved their condition. It also aids in memory enhancement and improved concentration. Shifting to a keto diet has also improved the sleeping habits of people who have insomnia.

Improves the condition of PCOS

Polycystic ovarian syndrome (PCOS) is a disease in which the ovaries develop so quickly and cysts shape. A high carbohydrate diet may aggravate the disorder. The ketogenic diet, on the other hand, lets women maintain hormonal equilibrium, weight reduction, and increased LH (luteinizing hormone) and FSH (follicle-stimulating hormone) levels in the body.

Different types of Ketogenic diets

Ketogenic diets are classified into many groups. These diets are both focused on the same ideals, which implies that ketosis is their primary target. The following are few variations of the diet:

The standard ketogenic diet (SKD)

This is the most popular form of diet, which consists of a low carbohydrate intake, a medium protein intake, and a high fat intake in the ratio of 1:4:15.

Targeted Ketogenic diet (TKD)

This plan is identical to the traditional ketogenic diet; but, on this diet, carbs

should only be progressively included whether you eat or work out.

The cyclical ketogenic diet (CKD)

This is yet another common diet that allows you to eat carbs only during certain periods. This diet includes a few days of ketosis accompanied by days of carbohydrate ingestion. Holding five ketogenic days a week accompanied by two carbohydrate days is a smart plan.

High-protein ketogenic diet

This diet emphasizes strong protein consumption, as the name implies. It's similar to the traditional ketogenic diet, but instead of fat, it emphasizes protein intake. The fat, protein, and carbohydrate ratios are now 12:7:1.

CHAPTER 2:

Keto Chaffles

A keto waffle is known as a chaffle. Since melted cheese is one of the key ingredients, it's called a chaffle rather than a waffle, and chaffles are cheese waffles. Waffles are usually produced with flour, while chaffles are made with eggs and cheese. It might sound strange, but it works! Chaffles are a fantastic way to get your waffle fix when on the keto diet.

Easiest Way to Produce Chaffles

Chaffles can be made in five simple steps using just a waffle making machine for flat chaffles and a waffle bowl maker for chaffle bowls.

Chaffles may only be made with two ingredients

- Cheese
- Eggs

To make a basic chaffle, follow the following simple steps--

- To start, preheat your waffle making machine until it is high enough.

- Meanwhile, in a bowl, whisk together the egg and cheese by hand until thoroughly combined.
- Cover the iron after pouring about a quarter or half of the mixture.
- Cook for 5 to 7 minutes, or until the chaffle is crispy.
- Place the chaffle on a plate and set it aside to cool before serving.

Tips to Make Chaffles

Preheat Well

Yeah, indeed! Preheating the waffle iron until usage appears self-evident. However, if you preheat the iron just slightly, the chaffles would not be as crispy as you might want. The best approach to preheat an iron before cooking is to make sure it's really hot.

Not-So-Cheesy

Do you want your chaffles to be less cheesy? Then add mozzarella cheese to the mix.

Not-So Eggy

If the scent of eggs in your chaffles scares you, consider using egg whites instead of egg yolks or whole eggs.

To Shred or Slice

When making chaffles, several recipes call for shredded cheese; however, sliced cheeses have crispier bits. Although it's best to use shredded cheese since it's more convenient, you can also use sliced cheese of about the same volume.

When using sliced cheeses, put two to four parts in the waffle iron, top with beaten eggs, and a few slices of cheese. Cook, wrapped, until crispy.

Shallower Irons

Using shallower waffle irons for crispier chaffles, and they cook better and quicker.

Layering

Don't overcrowd the waffle iron with batter. For properly done chaffles, use about a quarter and a half cups of total ingredients per batch.

Patience

Creating chaffles is a virtue. Enable the chaffles to hang in the iron for 5 to 7 minutes before serving for best outcomes.

No Peeking

Waiting seven minutes for the result of your squabbles isn't that much. You have a higher risk of ruining the chaffle by opening the iron and checking on it until it is done.

Crispy Cooling

Allowing the chaffles to cool more after moving to a plate is strongly suggested for optimal crispiness.

Easy Cleaning

Moist a paper towel and brush the iron's inner sections when it's still warm for the maximum clean-up. Please bear in mind that the iron should be warm, not hot!

Brush It

For a good cleaning, use a clean toothbrush to clean between the iron's teeth. While the iron is still warm, you should clean it with a dry, rough sponge.

CHAPTER 3:

Basic Chaffle Recipes

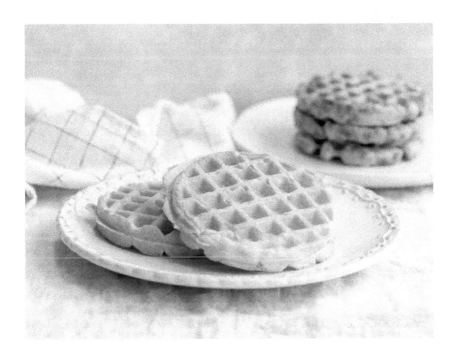

Chocolate Vanilla Chaffles

Preparation Time-5 minutes| Cook Time-5 minutes| Total
Time- 10 minutes| Servings-2| Difficulty-Easy

Nutritional Facts- Carbohydrates--23 g|Fat-3 g|Protein-4
g|Calories-134

Ingredients

- One egg
- One teaspoon of vanilla extract
- Two tablespoons of almond meal or flour
- Half cup shredded mozzarella cheese
- One tablespoon of granulated sweetener
- One tablespoon of sugar-free chocolate chips

Instructions

- Turn on the waffle making machine to heat and oil it with cooking spray.
- Mix all components in a bowl until combined.
- Introduce half of the batter into the waffle making machine.
- Cook for 2-minutes, then remove and repeat with the remaining batter.
- Top with more chips and favorite toppings.

Strawberry Chaffles

Preparation Time-5 minutes| Cook Time-10 minutes| Total Time- 15 minutes| Servings-2 | Difficulty-Easy

Nutritional Facts- Calories-69|Net Carb-1.6g|Fat-4.6g|Saturated Fat-2.2g| Carbohydrates- 1.9g| Dietary Fiber-0.3g| Sugar-1g|Protein-4.2 g

Ingredients

- A quarter cup of shredded Mozzarella cheese
- A quarter teaspoon organic baking powder
- Two fresh sliced and hulled strawberries
- One beaten organic egg
- One tablespoon of softened cream cheese
- One teaspoon of organic strawberry extract

Instructions

- Preheat mini waffle iron and then oil it.
- In a bowl, place all ingredients except strawberry slices and beat until well combined. Fold in the strawberry slices.
- Put a portion of the mixture into preheated waffle iron and cook for about minutes or until golden brown.
- Repeat with the remaining mixture. Serve warm.

Cinnamon Chaffles

Preparation Time-5 minutes| Cook Time-10 minutes| Total Time- 15 minutes| Servings-2 | Difficulty-Easy

Nutritional Facts- Calories 142| Net Carbohydrates- 2.1 g| Total Fat- 10.6 g| Saturated Fat-4 g |Cholesterol-106 mg| Sodium-122 mg| Total Carbohydrates- 4.1 g| Fiber-2 g| Sugar-0.3 g| Protein-7.7 g

Ingredients

- ¾ cup of shredded mozzarella cheese
- Two tablespoons of blanched almond flour
- Half teaspoon of ground cinnamon
- One beaten large organic egg
- Half tablespoon of melted unsalted butter
- Two tablespoons of Erythritol
- Half teaspoon of Psyllium husk powder
- Half teaspoon of organic vanilla extract
- A quarter teaspoon organic baking powder

For the topping

- ¾ teaspoon of ground cinnamon
- One teaspoon of powdered Erythritol

Instructions

- Preheat the waffle iron and then oil it.
- For chaffles, in a medium bowl, put all ingredients and with a fork, mix until well combined.

- Put a portion of the mixture into preheated waffle iron and cook for about 5 minutes.

- Repeat with the remaining mixture. Meanwhile, for topping, in a small bowl, mix the Erythritol and cinnamon.

- Place the chaffles onto serving plates and set them aside to cool slightly.

- Sprinkle with the cinnamon mixture and serve immediately.

Whipping Cream Chaffles

Preparation Time-5 minutes| Cook Time-10 minutes| Total Time- 15 minutes| Servings-2 | Difficulty-Easy

Nutritional Facts- Calories-112|Net Carb-1.8g|Fat-6.9g| Saturated Fat- 2.7g| Carbohydrates- 3.7g| Dietary Fiber-2.1g| Sugar-0.2g |Protein-10.9g

Ingredients

- One tablespoon heavy whipping cream
- Two tablespoons of Erythritol
- A quarter teaspoon of peanut butter extract
- One beaten organic egg
- Two tablespoons of sugar-free peanut butter powder
- A quarter teaspoon of organic baking powder

Instructions

- Preheat mini waffle iron and then oil it.
- Add all ingredients to a medium bowl and, with a fork, mix until well mixed.
- Put half of the mixture in the preheated waffle iron and cook until golden brown or around 4 minutes.
- Repeat with the mixture that remains. Serve it hot.

Light & Crispy Bacon-Egg Chaffles

Preparation Time-10 minutes| Cook Time-5 minutes| Total Time- 15 minutes| Servings-2 | Difficulty-Easy

Nutritional   Facts- Calories-320|Carbohydrates-2.9   g| Protein-21.5 g| Fat-24.3g

Ingredients

- Half cup of shredded cheese
- Fried eggs
- One large egg
- Thick-cut bacon
- Sliced cheese

Instructions

- Preheat your waffle making machine.
- Mix the egg and the shredded cheese together in a small mixing bowl. Stir until combined well.
- Onto the waffle making machine, add one half of the waffle batter. Cook until golden brown or 3-4 minutes. Repeat with the batter for the second half.
- Cook the bacon until crispy in a wide pan over medium heat. In the same pan, fry the egg over medium heat with One tablespoon of reserved bacon drippings.
- Cook until the doneness is needed. Assemble and enjoy the sandwich!

White Bread Keto Chaffle

Preparation Time-5 minutes| Cook Time-5 minutes| Total Time- 10 minutes| Servings-2 | Difficulty-Easy

Nutritional Facts- Calories-320| Carbohydrates-2.9 g| Protein-21.5 g| Fat-24.3g

Ingredients

- Melted cream cheese
- A quarter teaspoon of baking powder
- A Pinch of salt
- Two egg whites
- Two teaspoons of water
- A quarter cup of almond flour

Instructions

- Preheat the mini waffle making machine.
- Beat the egg whites with the cream cheese and water in a bowl.
- The next step is to add the baking powder, almond flour, salt and whisk until you have a smooth batter.
- Then, introduce half of the batter into the mini waffle making machine. Allow cooking for roughly 4 minutes or until you no longer see steam coming from the waffle making machine.
- Remove and allow to cool.

CHAPTER 4:

Breakfast Recipes

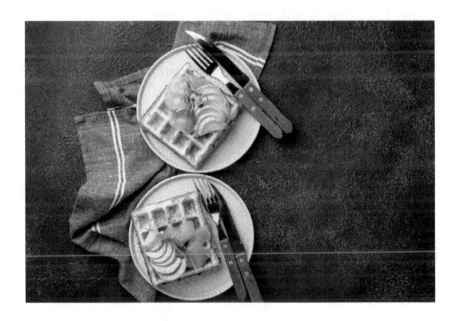

Blackberry Chaffles

Preparation Time-5 minutes| Cook Time-10 minutes| Total Time- 15 minutes| Servings-2 | Difficulty-Easy

Nutritional Facts- Calories-121|Net Carb-2.6g|Fat-7.5g|Saturated Fat-3.3g| Carbohydrates- 4.5g|Dietary Fiber-1.8g| Sugar-0.9g|Protein-8.9g

Ingredients

- 1/3 cup of shredded Mozzarella cheese
- One teaspoon of coconut flour
- ¾ teaspoon of powdered Erythritol
- A quarter teaspoon organic vanilla extract
- One tablespoon of fresh blackberries
- One beaten organic egg
- One teaspoon of softened cream cheese
- A quarter teaspoon of organic baking powder
- A quarter teaspoon of ground cinnamon
- Pinch of salt

Instructions

- Preheat mini waffle iron and then oil it.
- In a bowl, place all ingredients except for blackberries and beat until well combined. Fold in the blackberries.
- Put a portion of the mixture into preheated waffle iron and cook for about minutes or until golden brown.
- Repeat with the remaining mixture. Serve warm.

Morning Chaffles With Berries

Preparation Time-10 minutes| Cook Time-5 minutes| Total Time- 15 minutes| Servings-4 | Difficulty-Easy

Nutritional Facts- Protein-68kcal |Fat-163kcal |Carbohydrates- 12kcal

Ingredients

- One cup of shredded cheddar cheese

- A quarter cup of heavy cream

- One cup of egg whites

- A quarter cup of almond flour

For topping

- Four oz. of strawberries

- One oz. of feta cheese

- Four oz. of raspberries

- One oz. of keto chocolate flakes

Instructions

- Preheat your square waffle making machine and oil with cooking spray.

- In a small bowl, beat the white egg with the flour Add shredded cheese to the egg whites and flour mixture and mix well. Add cream and cheese to the egg mixture.

- Pour Chaffles batter in a waffle making machine and cover.

- Cook chaffles for about 4 minutes until crispy and brown. Carefully remove chaffles from the maker.

- Serve with berries, cheese, and chocolate on top. Enjoy!

Egg & Bacon Sandwich Chaffles

Preparation Time-6 minutes| Cook Time-20 minutes| Total Time- 26 minutes| Servings-4 | Difficulty-Easy

Nutritional Facts- Calories-197 |Total Fat-14.5g| Saturated Fat-4.1g| Cholesterol-2mg| Sodium-224g| Total Carbohydrates- 2.7g| Protein-12.9 g

Ingredients

For Chaffles

- Four tablespoons of almond flour
- One cup of shredded mozzarella cheese
- Two beaten large organic eggs
- One teaspoon of organic baking powder

For the Filling

- Four cooked bacon slices
- Four organic fried eggs

Instructions

- Preheat mini waffle iron and then oil it.
- In a medium bowl, put all ingredients and with a fork, mix thoroughly.
- Put a portion of the mixture into preheated waffle iron and cook for about 3–5 minutes.
- Repeat with the remaining mixture. Repeat with the remaining mixture.
- Serve each chaffle with filling ingredients.

Pumpkin & Psyllium Husk Chaffles

Preparation Time-8 minutes| Cook Time-16 minutes| Total Time- 24 minutes| Servings-2 | Difficulty-Easy

Nutritional Facts- Calories-221| Carb-0.6g|Fat-2.8g|Saturated Fat-1.1g| Carbohydrates- 0.8g| Dietary Fiber-0.2g| Sugar-0.4g|Protein-3.9g

Ingredients

- Half cup of shredded mozzarella cheese
- Two teaspoons of Erythritol
- 1/3 teaspoon of ground cinnamon
- Half teaspoon of organic vanilla extract
- Two organic eggs
- One tablespoon of homemade pumpkin puree
- Half teaspoon of psyllium husk powder
- Pinch of salt

Instructions

- Preheat mini waffle iron and then oil it.
- In a bowl, place all ingredients and beat until well combined.
- Place the quarter of the mixture into preheated waffle iron and cook for about 4 minutes or until golden brown.
- Repeat with the remaining mixture. Serve warm.

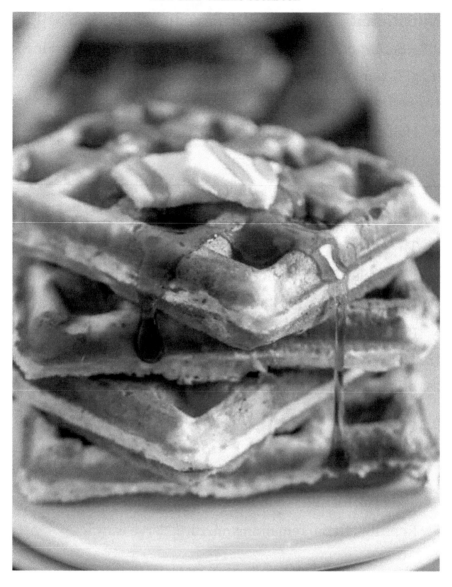

CHAPTER 5:

Lunch Recipes

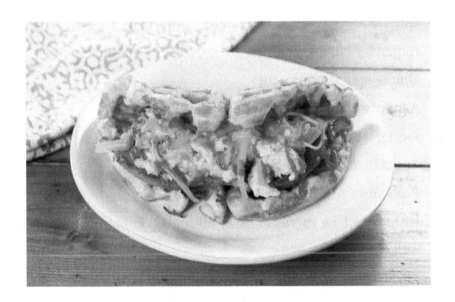

Chicken & Ham chaffles

Preparation Time-10 minutes| Cook Time-16 minutes| Total Time- 26 minutes| Servings-2 | Difficulty-Easy

Nutritional Facts- Calories-71|Net Carb-0.7g|Fat-4.2g|Saturated Fat-2g| Carbohydrates- 0.8g|Dietary Fiber-0.1g |Sugar-0.2g|Protein-7.4g

Ingredients

- One ounce of chopped sugar-free ham
- A quarter cup of chopped grass-fed cooked chicken
- One beaten organic egg
- A quarter cup of shredded mozzarella cheese
- A quarter cup of shredded swiss cheese

Instructions

- Preheat mini waffle iron and then oil it.
- Introduce to a medium bowl all ingredients and mix until well combined.
- Place ¼ of the mixture into preheated waffle iron and cook for about 4 minutes or until golden brown.
- Repeat with the remaining mixture. Serve warm.

Chicken & Zucchini Chaffles

Preparation Time-5 minutes| Cook Time-20 minutes| Total Time- 25 minutes| Servings-9 | Difficulty-Easy

Nutritional Facts- Calories-108|Net Carb-2g|Fat-6.9g| Saturated Fat-2.2g| Carbohydrates- 3.1g|Dietary Fiber-1.1g |Sugar-0.3g|Protein-8.8g

Ingredients

- Two cups of shredded and squeezed zucchini
- Two large organic eggs
- Half cup of shredded Cheddar cheese
- One teaspoon of organic baking powder
- Half teaspoon of onion powder
- Four ounces of chopped and cooked grass-fed chicken
- A quarter cup of chopped scallion
- Half cup of shredded mozzarella cheese
- Half cup of blanched almond flour
- Half teaspoon of garlic salt

Instructions

- Preheat the waffle iron and then oil it.
- Introduce to a medium bowl all ingredients and mix until well combined.
- Divide the mixture into nine portions.
- Place one portion of the mixture into preheated waffle iron and cook for about 2-3 minutes or until golden brown.
- Repeat with the remaining mixture. Serve warm.

Spinach & Artichoke Chicken Chaffle

Preparation Time-5 minutes| Cook Time-10 minutes| Total Time- 15 minutes| Servings-2| Difficulty-Easy

Nutritional Facts- Calories-320| Carbohydrates-2.9 g| Protein-21.5 g| Fat-24.3g

Ingredients

- 1/3 cup of chopped and cooked spinach
- 1/3 cup of shredded mozzarella cheese
- 1/3 cup of cooked and diced chicken
- 1/3 cup of chopped and marinated artichokes
- One ounce of softened cream cheese
- One egg
- A quarter teaspoon of garlic powder

Instructions

- Heat up your mini waffle making machine.
- Mix the egg, garlic powder, cream cheese, and mozzarella cheese in a small cup. Connect the artichoke, spinach, and chicken and combine well.
- Using your mini waffle making machine, add 1/3 of the batter and cook for 4 minutes. If it's still a little uncooked, leave it for another 2 minutes to cook.

- Then, to make a second chaffle, cook the remaining batter and then cook the third chaffle.
- Take it out of the pan after cooking and let it sit for 2 minutes. Immerse it in ranch dressing or sour cream.

Garlic Chicken Chaffle

Preparation Time-10 minutes| Cook Time-15 minutes| Total Time- 25 minutes| Servings-2 | Difficulty-Easy

Nutritional Facts- Calories-475| fat-29.5 g| Carbohydrates-7.2 g| sugar-0.4 |Protein-44.7 g|sodium-286 mg

Ingredients

For Batter

- Two cups of grated mozzarella cheese
- Two tablespoons of coconut flour
- Pepper and salt to taste
- Four eggs
- A quarter cup of almond flour
- Two and a half teaspoons of baking powder

For Garlic Chicken Topping

- Pepper and salt as per taste
- One pound of diced chicken
- One teaspoon of dried oregano
- Three tablespoons of butter
- Two minced garlic cloves

Other

- Two tablespoons of freshly chopped parsley
- Two tablespoons of cooking spray

Instructions

- Preheat the waffle making machine.

- Add the eggs, grated mozzarella cheese, almond flour, coconut flour and baking powder to a bowl and season with pepper and salt. Mix until just combined.

- Spray the waffle making machine with cooking spray to prevent the chaffles from sticking. Add a few tablespoons of the batter to the preheated and oiled waffle making machine.

- Cover and cook for about 7 minutes, depending on your waffle making machine.

- Repeat with the rest of the batter.

- Meanwhile, melt the butter in a non-stick pan over medium heat. Season the chicken with pepper and salt and dried oregano and mix in the minced garlic. Cook the chicken while stirring periodically for about 10 minutes.

- Serve each chaffle with a topping of the garlic chicken mixture and sprinkle some freshly chopped parsley on top.

Keto Chaffle Taco Shells

Preparation Time-5 minutes| Cook Time-20 minutes| Total Time- 25 minutes| Servings-5 | Difficulty-Easy

Nutritional   Facts- Calories-113kcal |Protein-8g| Carbohydrates- 1g |Fat-9g

Ingredients

- One cup of taco blend cheese
- A quarter teaspoon of taco seasoning
- One tablespoon of almond flour
- Two eggs

Instructions

- Combine the almond flour, taco cheese mix, eggs, and taco seasoning in a dish using a fork.

- Introduce one and a half tablespoons of taco chaffle batter at a time to the waffle making machine| cook 4 minutes of chaffle batter in the waffle making machine.

- Remove the waffle making machine's taco chaffle shell and drape it over the side of a bowl. Keep making taco chaffle shells until you're out of the batter.

- Then fill the taco shells with taco meat, and enjoy your favorite toppings.

CHAPTER 6:

Dinner Recipes

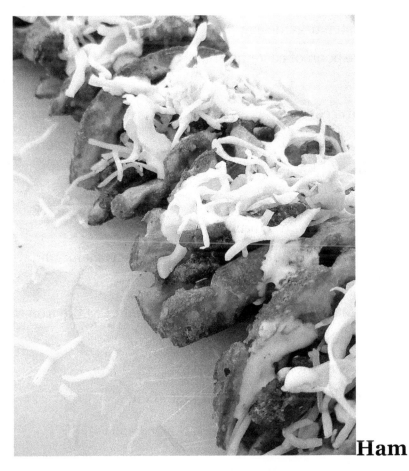

Ham
Sandwich Chaffles

Preparation Time-6 minutes| Cook Time-8 minutes| Total Time- 14 minutes| Servings-2 | Difficulty- Easy

Nutritional Facts- Calories 111|Net Carbohydrates- 3.7g| Total Fa- 8.7g |Saturated Fat-3.4g|Cholesterol-114mg|Total Carbohydrates- 5.5g|Protein 13.9g

Ingredients

- Half cup of shredded Monterrey Jack cheese
- Pinch of garlic powder
- One beaten organic egg
- One teaspoon of coconut flour

Filling

- Two lettuce leaves
- One small sliced tomato
- Two sugar-free ham slices

Instructions

- Preheat mini waffle iron and then oil it.
- For chaffles, in a medium bowl, put all ingredients and with a fork, mix thoroughly.
- Put a portion of the mixture into preheated waffle iron and cook for about 3–4 minutes.
- Repeat with the remaining mixture.
- Serve each chaffle with filling ingredients.

Barbecue Chaffle

Preparation Time-10 minutes| Cook Time-8 minutes| Total Time- 18 minutes| Servings-2 | Difficulty- Easy

Nutritional Facts- Calories-295|Total Fat-23 g| Saturated Fat-13 g |Cholesterol-223 mg |Sodium-414 mg |Potassium-179 mg |Total Carbohydrates-2 g |Dietary Fiber-1 g| Protein-20 g| Total Sugars-1g

Ingredients

- Half cup of shredded cheddar cheese
- A quarter teaspoon of baking powder
- One beaten egg
- Half teaspoon barbecue sauce

Instructions

- Plugin your waffle making machine to preheat.
- Mix all the ingredients in a bowl.
- Introduce half of the mixture to your waffle making machine.
- Cover and cook for minutes.
- Repeat the same steps for the next barbecue chaffle, and then serve warm.

Chicken & Jalapeño Chaffles

Preparation Time-6 minutes| Cook Time-10 minutes| Total Time- 16 minutes| Servings-2 | Difficulty- Easy

Nutritional Facts- Calories-170|Net Carb-0.9g|Fat-9.9g|Saturated Fat-5.2g| Carbohydrates- 0.1g|Dietary Fiber-2| Sugar-0.5g|Protein-8.6g

Ingredients

- One beaten organic egg
- Two tablespoons of shredded parmesan cheese
- One small chopped jalapeño pepper
- 1/8 teaspoon of garlic powder
- Half cup of grass-fed cooked and chopped chicken
- A quarter cup of shredded cheddar cheese
- One teaspoon of softened cream cheese
- 1/8 teaspoon of onion powder

Instructions

- Preheat mini waffle iron and then oil it.
- Introduce to a medium bowl all ingredients and mix until well combined.
- Put a portion of the mixture into preheated waffle iron and cook for about 4-5 minutes or until golden brown.
- Repeat with the remaining mixture. Serve warm.

CHAPTER 7:

Sweet Recipes

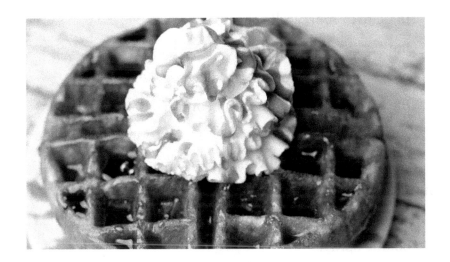

Banana Nut Chaffle

Preparation Time-5 minutes| Cook Time-10 minutes| Total Time- 15 minutes| Servings-1 | Difficulty-Easy

Nutritional Facts- Carbohydrates-2 g|Fat-g|Protein-8 g|Calories-119

Ingredients

- One tablespoon of softened cream cheese
- Half cup of mozzarella cheese
- One egg
- One tablespoon of sugar-free cheesecake pudding
- One tablespoon of monk fruit confectioners' sweetener
- A quarter teaspoon of banana extract toppings of choice
- A quarter teaspoon of vanilla extract

Instructions

- Turn on the waffle making machine to heat and oil it with cooking spray.
- Beat egg in a small bowl. Add remaining ingredients and mix until well incorporated.
- Add one-half of the batter to the waffle making machine and cook for minutes until golden brown.
- Remove the chaffle and add the other half of the batter. Top with your optional toppings and serve warm!

Mocha Chaffles

Preparation Time-5 minutes| Cook Time-10 minutes| Total Time- 15 minutes| Servings-3 | Difficulty-Easy

Nutritional Facts- Calories-83|Net Carb-1g|Fat-7.5g|Saturated Fat-4.6g| Carbohydrates- 1.5g|Dietary Fiber-0.5g |Sugar-0.3g|Protein-2.7g

Ingredients

- One tablespoon of cacao powder
- A quarter teaspoon of organic baking powder
- One tablespoon of mayonnaise
- One beaten organic egg
- One tablespoon of Erythritol
- Two tablespoons of softened cream cheese
- A quarter teaspoon of instant coffee powder
- One teaspoon of organic vanilla extract
- A Pinch of salt

Instructions

- Preheat mini waffle iron and then oil it.
- In a medium bowl, place all ingredients and with a fork, mix until well combined.
- Place half of the mixture into preheated waffle iron and cook for about 2½-3 minutes or until golden brown.
- Repeat with the remaining mixture. Serve warm.

Chaffles With Strawberry Frosty

Preparation Time-7 minutes| Cook Time-5 minutes| Total Time- 12 minutes| Servings-3 | Difficulty-Easy

Nutritional Facts- Protein-13g |Fat-69g| Carbohydrates-18g

Ingredients

- Half cup of Heavy cream
- One cup of frozen strawberries
- One teaspoon of stevia
- Three keto chaffles
- One scoop of protein powder

Instructions

- Mix all the above ingredients in a mixing bowl except the chaffles.
- Pour mixture in silicone molds and freeze in a freezer for about 4 hours to set.
- Once frosty is set, top on keto chaffles and enjoy!

Blueberry Cream Cheese Chaffles

Preparation Time-5 minutes| Cook Time-10 minutes| Total Time- 15 minutes| Servings-2 | Difficulty-Easy

Nutritional Facts- Calories-120|Net Carb-1.9g|Fat-9.6g|Saturated Fat-2.2g| Carbohydrates- 3.1g|Dietary Fiber-1.3g |Sugar-1g|Protein-3.2g

Ingredients

- One tablespoon of softened cream cheese
- A quarter teaspoon organic baking powder
- Four to six fresh blueberries
- One beaten organic egg
- Three tablespoons of almond flour
- One teaspoon of organic blueberry extract

Instructions

- Preheat mini waffle iron and then oil it.
- In a bowl, place all the ingredients except blueberries and beat until well combined. Fold in the blueberries. Divide the mixture into five portions.
- Place one portion of the mixture into preheated waffle iron and cook for about 3-4 minutes or until golden brown.
- Repeat with the remaining mixture. Serve warm.

Apple Pie Chaffle

Preparation Time-10 minutes| Cook Time-10 minutes| Total Time- 20 minutes| Servings-2 | Difficulty-Easy

Nutritional Facts- Fat-7.8g|Carbohydrate-10g| Sugars-12.1g| Protein-5.4g

Ingredients

- One tablespoon of almond flour
- One tablespoon of heavy whipping cream
- One tablespoon of granulated Swerve
- One beaten egg
- One big finely chopped apple
- One teaspoon of cinnamon
- Half teaspoon of vanilla extract
- A quarter tablespoon of sugar-free maple syrup
- 1/3 cup of mozzarella cheese

Instructions

- Plug the waffle making machine and preheat it. Spray it with non-stick spray.
- In a large mixing bowl, combine the swerve, almond flour, mozzarella, cinnamon and chopped apple. Add the eggs, vanilla extract and heavy whipping cream.
- Mix until all the ingredients are well combined.
- Fill the waffle making machine with the batter and spread out the batter to the edges of the waffle making machine to all the holes on it. Cover and cook for about 4 minutes.

- After the cooking cycle, remove the chaffle from the waffle making machine.
- Serve and top with maple syrup.

Cinnamon Pumpkin Chaffles

Preparation Time-8 minutes| Cook Time-16 minutes| Total Time- 24 minutes| Servings-2 | Difficulty-Easy

Nutritional Facts- Calories- 321|Net Carb-1.4g|Fat-4g|Saturated Fat-1.3g| Carbohydrates- 2.5g|Dietary Fiber-1.1g |Sugar-0.6g|Protein-4.3 g

Ingredients

- 2/3 cup of shredded mozzarella cheese
- Three teaspoons of almond flour
- Two teaspoons of ground cinnamon
- Two organic eggs
- Three tablespoons of sugar-free pumpkin puree
- Two teaspoons of granulated Erythritol

Instructions

- Preheat mini waffle iron and then oil it.
- Add all ingredients to a medium bowl and, with a fork, mix until well mixed.
- Put half of the mixture in the preheated waffle iron and cook until golden brown or around 4 minutes.
- Repeat with the mixture that remains. Serve it hot.

Fudgy Chocolate Chaffles

Preparation Time-5 minutes| Cook Time-10 minutes| Total Time- 15 minutes| Servings-2 | Difficulty-Easy

Nutritional Facts- Carbohydrates- 5g |Protein-7g |Fat-7g|Calories-109kcal

Ingredients

- Two tablespoons of shredded mozzarella cheese
- Two tablespoons of Lakanto monk fruit powder
- One teaspoon of heavy whipping cream
- One egg
- Two tablespoons of cocoa
- One teaspoon of coconut flour
- A quarter teaspoon of baking powder
- A pinch of salt
- A quarter teaspoon of vanilla extract

Instructions

- Switch on the chaffle or waffle making machine.
- Lightly oil or use cooking spray.
- Combine every ingredient in a small bowl.
- Pour 1/2 of the batter into the waffle making machine.
- Close the lid of the waffle making machine and cook for 4 minutes. Cautiously remove the chaffle from the waffle making machine. Repeat the above steps.
- Serve with sugar-free strawberry ice cream or whipped topping without sugar.

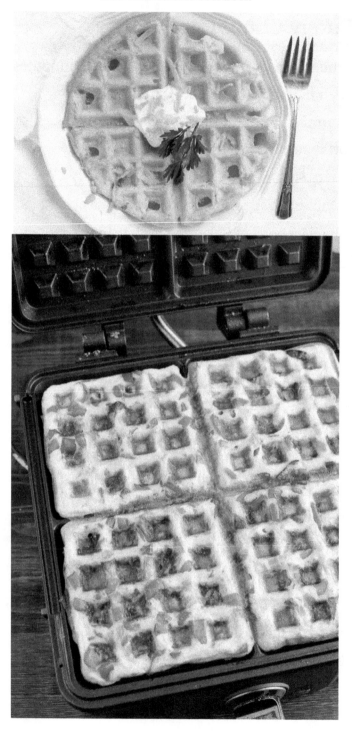

CHAPTER 8:

Savory Recipes

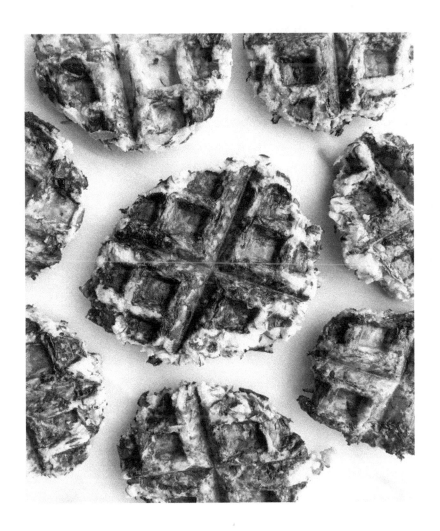

Scallion Chaffles

Preparation Time-6 minute| Cook Time-8 minutes| Total Time- 14 minutes| Servings-2 | Difficulty- Easy

Nutritional Facts- Calories-52 |Net Carb-0.7g|Fat-3.8g|Saturated Fat-1.5g|Carbohydrates- 0.8g|Dietary Fiber-0.7g| Sugar-0.3g|Protein-4.8g

Ingredients

- Half cup of shredded mozzarella cheese
- Half teaspoon Italian seasoning
- One beaten organic egg
- One tablespoon of chopped scallion

Instructions

- Preheat mini waffle iron and then oil it.
- Introduce to a medium bowl all ingredients and mix until well combined.
- Put a portion of the mixture in the preheated waffle iron and cook until golden brown or around 4 minutes.
- Repeat with the mixture that remains. Serve it hot.

Parmesan Garlic Chaffle

Preparation Time-6 minute| Cook Time-5 minutes| Total Time- 11 minutes| Servings-2 | Difficulty- Easy

Nutritional Facts- Carbohydrates-5 g|Fat-33 g|Protein-19 g|Calories-385

Ingredients

- Two tablespoons of butter
- Two tablespoons of almond flour
- Two large eggs
- One tablespoon of minced fresh garlic
- One oz of cubed cream cheese
- One teaspoon of baking soda
- One teaspoon of dried chives
- ¾ cup of shredded mozzarella cheese
- Half cup of shredded parmesan cheese

Instructions

- Heat cream cheese and butter in a saucepan over medium-low until melted.
- Add garlic and cook, stirring, for minutes. Turn on the waffle making machine to heat and oil it with cooking spray.
- In a small mixing bowl, whisk together flour and baking soda, then set aside.
- In a separate bowl, beat eggs for 1 minute 30 seconds on high, then add in cream cheese mixture and beat for 60 seconds more.

- Add flour mixture, chives, and cheeses to the bowl and stir well. Add a quarter cup of batter to the waffle making machine.

- Close and cook for 4 minutes, until golden brown. Repeat for the remaining batter. Add favorite toppings and serve.

Pepperoni Chaffles

Preparation Time-5 minute| Cook Time-5 minutes| Total Time- 10 minutes| Servings-2 | Difficulty- Easy

Nutritional Facts- Calories-119|Net Carb-2.4g|Fat-7.3g|Saturated Fat-3g| Carbohydrates- 2.7g|Dietary Fiber-0.3g |Sugar-0.9g|Protein-10.3 g

Ingredients

- Half cup of shredded mozzarella cheese
- One beaten organic egg
- Two tablespoons of a chopped turkey pepperoni slice
- A quarter teaspoon of Italian seasoning
- One tablespoon sugar-free pizza sauce

Instructions

- Preheat the waffle iron and then oil it.
- Introduce in a bowl all the ingredients and mix well.
- Place the mixture into preheated waffle iron and cook for about 5 minutes or until golden brown.
- Serve warm.

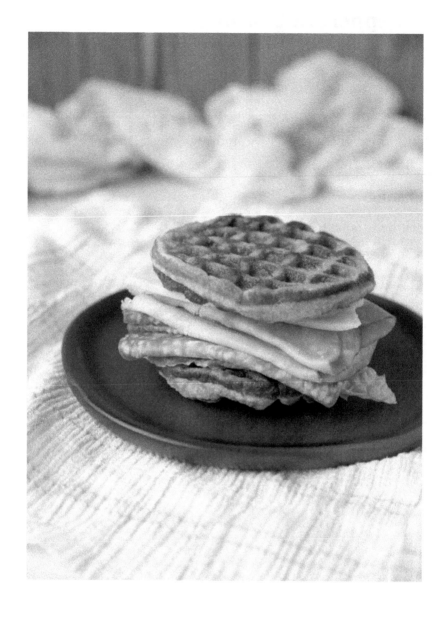

CHAPTER 9:

Fancy Vegetarian Recipes

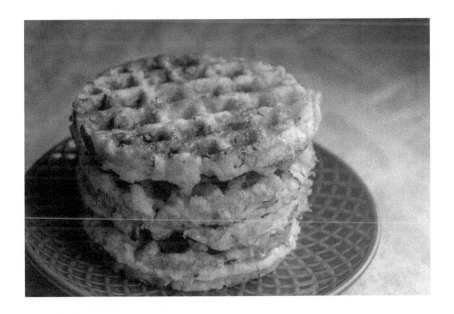

Zucchini & Onion Chaffles

Preparation Time-10 minutes| Cook Time-15 minutes| Total Time- 25 minutes| Servings-2 | Difficulty- Easy

Nutritional Facts- Calories-92|Net Carb-2g|Fat-5.3g|Saturated Fat-2.3g| Carbohydrates- 3.5g|Dietary Fiber-0.9g |Sugar-1.8g|Protein-8.6g

Ingredients

- Half cup of grated and squeezed onion
- Two cups of grated and squeezed zucchini
- Two organic eggs
- Half cup of grated Parmesan cheese
- Half cup of shredded Mozzarella cheese

Instructions

- Preheat the waffle iron and then oil it.
- Introduce to a medium bowl all ingredients and mix until well combined.
- Place ¼ of the mixture into preheated waffle iron and cook for about 4 minutes or until golden brown.
- Repeat with the remaining mixture. Serve warm.

Zucchini Chaffles With Peanut Butter

Preparation Time-10 minutes| Cook Time-5 minutes| Total Time- 15 minutes| Servings-2 | Difficulty- Easy

Nutritional Facts- Protein-88kcal| Fat-69kcal| Carbohydrates- 12kcal

Ingredients

- One egg beaten
- A quarter cup of shredded mozzarella cheese
- Half teaspoon of salt
- Two tablespoons of peanut butter
- One cup of grated zucchini
- Half cup of shredded parmesan cheese
- One teaspoon of dried basil
- Half teaspoon of black pepper

Instructions

- Sprinkle salt over zucchini and let it sit for a minute.
- Squeeze out water from zucchini. Beat egg with zucchini, basil, salt, mozzarella cheese, and pepper.
- Sprinkle ½ of the parmesan cheese over preheated waffle making machine and pour zucchini batter over it.
- Sprinkle the remaining cheese over it. Cover. Cook zucchini chaffles for about 4-8 minutes.

- Remove chaffles from the maker and repeat with the remaining batter.
- Serve with peanut butter on top, and enjoy!

Garlic and Spinach Chaffles

Preparation Time-10 minutes| Cook Time-5 minutes| Total Time- 15 minutes| Servings-2 | Difficulty- Easy

Nutritional Facts- Protein-88kcal |Fat-69kcal |Carbohydrates- 12kcal

Ingredients

- One teaspoon of Italian spice
- Half teaspoon of Vanilla
- One teaspoon of baking soda
- One cup of egg whites
- Two teaspoons of coconut flour
- One teaspoon of baking powder
- One cup of grated mozzarella cheese
- One cup of chopped spinach
- Half teaspoon of garlic powder

Instructions

- Switch on your square waffle making machine. Spray with non-stick spray.
- Beat egg whites with beater until fluffy and white.
- Add pumpkin puree, pumpkin pie spice, coconut flour in egg whites and beat again.
- Stir in the cheese, powder, garlic powder, baking soda, and powder. Sprinkle chopped spinach on a waffle making machine.

- Pour the batter into the waffle making machine over chopped spinach. Close the maker and cook for about 4-5 minutes. Remove chaffles from the maker.
- Serve hot and enjoy!

CHAPTER 10:

Easy Vegan Recipes

~ 68 ~

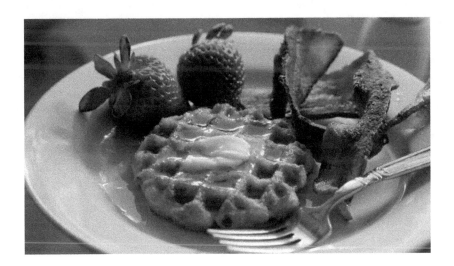

Fruity Vegan Chaffles

Preparation Time-5 minutes| Cook Time-5 minutes| Total Time- 10 minutes| Servings-2 | Difficulty- Easy

Nutritional Facts- Protein-32g |Fat-63g |Carbohydrates- 5g

Ingredients

- Two tablespoons of warm water
- Two tablespoons of strawberry puree
- A pinch of salt
- One tablespoon of chia seeds
- A quarter cup of low carb vegan cheese
- Two tablespoons of Greek yogurt

Instructions

- Preheat mini waffle making machine to medium-high heat.
- Mix chia seeds and water and let it stand for few minutes to be thickened.
- Mix the rest of the ingredients in a chia seed egg and mix well. Spray waffle machine with cooking spray.
- Introduce vegan waffle batter into the center of the waffle iron.
- Cover and cook chaffles for about 3-5 minutes.
- Once cooked, remove from the maker and serve with berries on top.

CHAPTER 11:

Meat Recipes

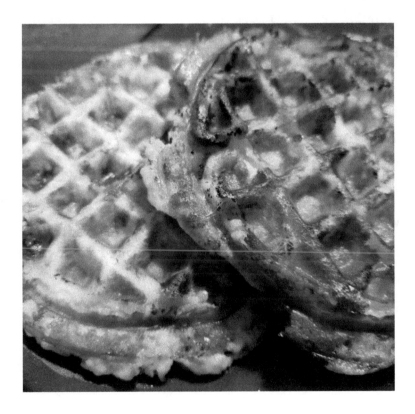

Pork Rind Chaffles

Preparation Time-6 minute| Cook Time-10 minutes| Total Time- 16 minutes| Servings-2 | Difficulty- Easy

Nutritional Facts- Calories-91|Net Carb-0.3g|Fat-5.9g|Saturated Fat-2.3g| Carbohydrates- 0.3g| Dietary Fiber-0g|Sugar-0.2g|Protein-9.2 g

Ingredients

- Half cup of ground pork rinds
- Pinch of salt
- One beaten organic egg
- 1/3 cup of shredded mozzarella cheese

Instructions

- Preheat mini waffle iron and then oil it.
- Introduce to a medium bowl all ingredients and mix until well combined.
- Put a portion of the mixture in the preheated waffle iron and cook until golden brown or around 5 minutes.
- Repeat with the remaining mixture. Serve warm.

Beef Chaffle Tower

Preparation Time-10 minutes| Cook Time-15 minutes| Total Time- 25 minutes| Servings-2 | Difficulty- Easy

Nutritional Facts- Calories-412| fat-25 g| Carbohydrates-1.8 g| sugar-0.5 g| Protein-43.2 g| sodium-256 m g

Ingredients

For the chaffle batter

- Two cups of grated mozzarella cheese
- Four eggs
- Pepper and salt to taste
- One teaspoon of Italian seasoning
- Two tablespoons of almond flour

For the Beef

- One pound of beef tenderloin
- Two tablespoons of butter
- Pepper and salt as per taste
- Two tablespoons of cooking spray
- One teaspoon of chili flakes

Instructions

- Preheat the waffle making machine.
- Add the eggs, grated mozzarella cheese, pepper and salt, almond flour and Italian seasoning to a bowl. Mix until everything is fully combined.
- Brush the preheated waffle making machine with cooking spray and add a few tablespoons of the batter.

- Cover and cook for about 7 minutes, depending on your waffle making machine.

- Meanwhile, heat the butter in a non-stick frying pan and season the beef tenderloin with pepper and salt and chili flakes. Cook the beef tenderloin for about 5–minutes on each side.

- When serving, assemble the chaffle tower by placing one chaffle on a plate, a layer of diced beef tenderloin, another chaffle, another layer of beef, and so on until you finish with the chaffles and beef.

- Serve and enjoy.

CHAPTER 12:

Festive Recipes

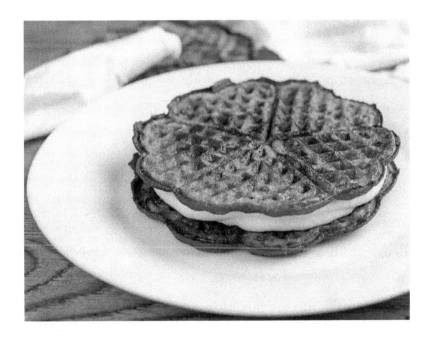

Pecan Pumpkin Chaffle

Preparation Time-10 minute| Cook Time-15 minutes| Total Time- 25 minutes| Servings-2| Difficulty- Easy

Nutritional Facts- Calories-121|Fat-9.2g|Carbohydrates-5.7g| sugar-3.3g| protein-6.7g| cholesterol-86 mg

Ingredients

- Two tablespoons of chopped and toasted pecans
- One teaspoon of erythritol
- One egg
- Two tablespoons of almond flour
- A quarter teaspoon of pumpkin pie spice
- Half cup of grated mozzarella cheese
- One tablespoon of pumpkin puree

Instructions

- Preheat your waffle making machine.
- Beat egg in a small bowl. Add remaining ingredients and mix well.
- Spray waffle making machine with cooking spray.
- Introduce half batter in the hot waffle making machine and cook for minutes or until golden brown.
- Repeat with the remaining batter. Serve and enjoy.

Pumpkin Chaffle With Frosting

Preparation Time-10 minute| Cook Time-15 minutes| Total Time- 25 minutes| Servings-2 | Difficulty- Easy

Nutritional Facts- Calories-99|Fat-7g|carbohydrates-3.6g| sugar-0.6g| protein-5.6g| cholesterol-97 mg

Ingredients

- One tablespoon of sugar-free pumpkin puree
- Half cup of shredded mozzarella cheese
- One lightly beaten egg
- A quarter teaspoon of pumpkin pie spice

For frosting

- Half teaspoon of vanilla
- Two tablespoons of softened cream cheese
- Two tablespoons of Swerve

Instructions

- Preheat your waffle making machine. Add egg in a bowl and whisk well.
- Add pumpkin puree, pumpkin pie spice, and cheese and stir well.
- Spray waffle making machine with cooking spray.
- Pour 1/2 of the batter into the hot waffle making machine and cook for 3-4 minutes or until golden brown.
- Repeat with the remaining batter.
- In a small bowl, mix all frosting ingredients until smooth.
- Add frosting on top of hot chaffles and serve.

Thanksgiving Pumpkin Latte with Chaffles

Preparation Time-10 minute| Cook Time-5 minutes| Total Time- 15 minutes| Servings-2 | Difficulty- Easy

Nutritional Facts- Protein-16g|Fat-259 g |Carbohydrates-29g

Ingredients

- Two tablespoons of Heavy cream
- One teaspoon of stevia
- 3/4 cup of unsweetened coconut milk
- Two tablespoons of pumpkin puree
- A quarter teaspoon of pumpkin spice
- A quarter cup of espresso
- A quarter teaspoon of Vanilla extract

For the toppings

- Two scoops of whipped cream
- Two basic heart-shaped chaffles
- A quarter teaspoon of pumpkin spice

Instructions

- Mix all recipe ingredients in mug and microwave for few minutes.
- Pour the latte into a serving glass.
- Top with a heavy cream scoop, pumpkin spice, and chaffle. Serve and enjoy!

CHAPTER 13:

Chaffle Cake Recipes

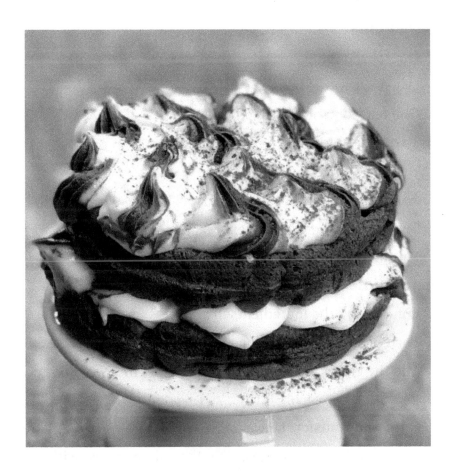

Banana Nut Muffin

Preparation Time-6 minutes| Cook Time-12 minutes| Total Time-18 minutes| Servings-2 | Difficulty-Easy

Nutritional Facts- Calories-169|Total Fat 14gSaturated Fat-4.6g|Cholesterol-99mg|Sodium-98mg|Potassium-343mg|Total Carbohydrate-5.6g|Dietary Fiber- 2g|Protein-5g|Total Sugars-0.6g

Ingredients

- One oz. of cream cheese
- One teaspoon of banana extract
- One teaspoon of baking powder
- Two tablespoons of chopped walnuts
- One egg
- A quarter cup of shredded mozzarella cheese
- Two tablespoons of sweetener
- Four tablespoons of almond flour

Instructions

- Combine all the ingredients in a bowl.
- Turn on the waffle making machine.
- Add the batter to the waffle making machine. Seal and cook for minutes.
- Open and transfer the waffle to a plate.
- Let cool for 2 minutes. Do the same steps with the remaining mixture.

CHAPTER 14:

Special Chaffle Recipes

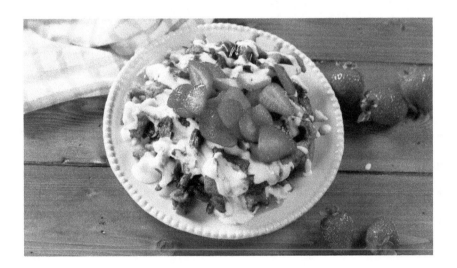

Pumpkin Cream Cheese Chaffles

Preparation Time-5 minute| Cook Time-10 minutes| Total Time- 15 minutes| Servings-2 | Difficulty- Easy

Nutritional Facts- Calories-110|Net Carb-2.5g|Fat-4.3g|Saturated Fat-1g|Carbohydrates- 3.3g|Dietary Fiber-0.8g| Sugar-1g|Protein-5.2g

Ingredients

- Half cup of shredded mozzarella cheese
- Two teaspoons of heavy cream
- One tablespoon of almond flour
- Half teaspoon of pumpkin pie spice
- One teaspoon of organic vanilla extract
- One beaten organic egg
- One and a half tablespoons of sugar-free pumpkin puree
- One teaspoon of softened cream cheese
- One tablespoon of Erythritol
- Half teaspoon of organic baking powder

Instructions

- Preheat mini waffle iron and then oil it.
- In a medium bowl, place all ingredients and with a fork, mix until well combined.
- Put a portion of the mixture into preheated waffle iron and cook for about 5 minutes or until golden brown.
- Repeat with the remaining mixture. Serve warm.

Chocolate Chips Lemon Chaffles

Preparation Time-8 minute| Cook Time-8 minutes| Total Time- 16 minutes| Servings-2| Difficulty- Easy

Nutritional Facts- Calories-235|Net Carb-1g|Fat-4.8g|Saturated Fat-2.3g| Carbohydrates- 1.5g|Dietary Fiber-0.5g| Sugar-0.3g| Protein-4.3g

Ingredients

- Half cup of shredded mozzarella cheese
- Half teaspoon of organic vanilla extract
- Half teaspoon of psyllium husk powder
- Two organic eggs
- ¾ teaspoon of organic lemon extract
- Two teaspoons of Erythritol
- Pinch of salt
- A quarter teaspoon of finely grated lemon zest
- One tablespoon of 70% dark chocolate chips

Instructions

- Preheat mini waffle iron and then oil it. In a bowl, place all ingredients except chocolate chips and lemon zest and beat until well combined.
- Gently fold in the chocolate chips and lemon zest.
- Place a quarter of the mixture into preheated waffle iron and cook for about minutes or until golden brown.
- Repeat with the remaining mixture. Serve warm.

Ube Chaffles With Ice Cream

Preparation Time-5 minutes| Cook Time-10 minutes| Total Time- 15 minutes| Servings-2 | Difficulty- Easy

Nutritional Facts- Calories65Kcal| Fats-16 g|Carbohydrates-7 g|Protein-22 g

Ingredients

- One tablespoon of whipped cream cheese
- One egg
- 1/3 cup of shredded mozzarella cheese
- Two tablespoons of sweetener
- Three drops of ube or pandan extract
- Keto ice cream
- Half teaspoon of baking powder

Instructions

- Add in 2 or 3 drops of ube extract, mix until creamy and smooth.
- Introduce half of the butter mixture in the mini waffle making machine and cook for about 5 minutes.
- Repeat the same steps with the remaining batter mixture. Top with keto ice cream and enjoy.

Conclusion

You should even hold the chaffles in the refrigerator. If you want to have chaffle meals in your regular diet, you might want to invest in one. Chaffle is an ideal way to relieve all of the hunger pangs.

We've been imaginative with the chaffle in this book, and we've included a number of recipes.

You will be able to follow your diet more easily now that you recognize the keto diet and how the chaffle will function as one of the better bread alternatives.

These book-recommended chaffle recipes are delectable and will make your mouth water.

This book has shown you how to fulfill your cravings when keeping low carb, whether you're searching for savory snacks, sweet foods, burgers, tacos, or sandwiches.

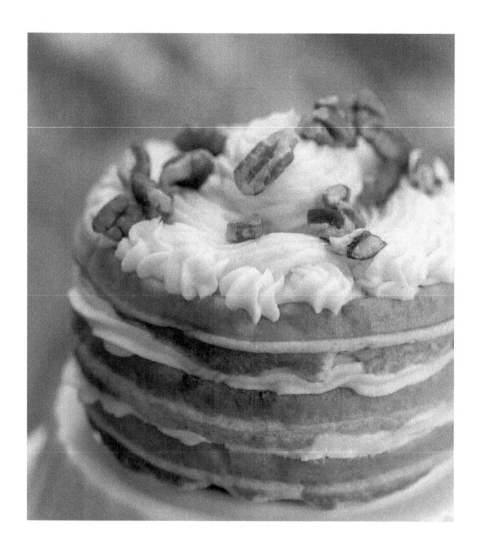

CPSIA information can be obtained
at www.ICGtesting.com
Printed in the USA
LVHW050342210621
690733LV00003B/214